OUTDOOR
SURVIVAL

A GUIDE TO STAYING SAFE OUTSIDE

Adventure Skills Guides

PERSEVERE IN THE WILDERNESS

T0166277

Adventure Skills Guides

This Adventure Skills Guide is a simple, straightforward resource about staying safe during an outdoor survival situation. It distills critical lessons gleaned from real-world survival scenarios into easy-to-digest tips. Whether you're hiking trails in the big woods of Minnesota or making camp in Colorado, the information in this guide will see you home.

Although the information is concise, it is also thorough. All steps in a survival scenario, from creating shelters and fire to signaling and moving, are covered. Also explained is what to de-prioritize, because doing nothing is always better than making the situation worse.

While this guide is designed for quick reference in high-stress conditions, it's advisable you read it ahead of time. Preparedness goes a long way, and it's not always about gear. Being mentally prepared for an unfortunate circumstance should be the first step, not the last.

BENJAMIN SOBIECK

Benjamin Sobieck is a former editor of *Living Ready* magazine, a publication dedicated to preparedness. His credits have also appeared in *BLADE, Gun Digest, Deer & Deer Hunting, Turkey & Turkey Hunting, Trapper & Predator Caller,* and *Tactical Gear,* among others. He lives in Minnesota.

Cover and book design by Lora Westberg
Edited by Brett Ortler

Cover image: **SF photo/shutterstock.com; Christos Siatos/shutterstock.com**

All images copyrighted.

Photos courtesy of: **Ben Sobieck:** 10, 18

Used under license from Shutterstock.com
AdrianH123: 11 bottom; **Asmiana:** 23; **robert cicchetti:** 11 middle; **Creation:** outside flap; **Ervin-Edward:** 25; **Salienko Evgenii:** 8; **Fotovika:** 22; **frantic00:** 23; **Geartooth Productions:** 9; **Henry Hazboun:** 9; **Zachary Hoover:** 11 top; **Burdun Illiya:** 24; **Mikhail Ivannikov:** 16; **Melissa King:** 14; **klyots:** 13; **Library of Congress, Public Domain:** Intro; **Little Noom:** 20; **Lizard:** 19; **Jaoslav Machacek:** 26; **Stanislav Makhalov:** 17; **Masonjar:** 4; **Zanna Pesnina:** 26; **LianeM:** outside flap (main); **Picture Maker:** 7; **PRESSLAB:** 6, 16; **Realstock:** 12; **sydeen:** 15; **This servants heart:** 13; **zlikovec:** 4

10 9 8 7 6 5 4

Outdoor Survival: A Guide to Staying Safe Outside
Copyright © 2019 by Benjamin Sobieck
Published by Adventure Publications, an imprint of AdventureKEEN
310 Garfield Street South, Cambridge, Minnesota 55008
(800) 678-7006
www.adventurepublications.net
All rights reserved
Printed in China
ISBN 978-1-59193-820-0 (pbk.)

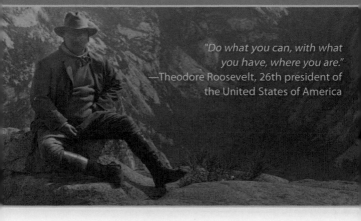

"Do what you can, with what you have, where you are."
—Theodore Roosevelt, 26th president of the United States of America

Good News Since you're reading this guide, one of two things happened: you're up the proverbial creek without a paddle, or you're getting a head start should you find yourself in a survival situation later on. In either case, I have good news: you're already doing things right. Most of survival has nothing to do with gear, guts, or grunt work. It's a mental game, and you're competing against yourself. Set your mind right with this guide, and the rest will follow.

The Goal Is to Be Rescued, Not to Be Rambo Let's get this out of the way right now: *your goal is to be rescued.* The best thing you can do is to sit tight, avoid anything dangerous, take care of your essential needs, and make yourself as easy to find as possible. It doesn't matter if you're in a tight spot for a couple of hours or a couple of days. The strategy remains the same.

Because no survival guide can predict what will happen until help arrives, the information in this guide is simple. Why? Simplicity equals versatility. You'll understand what this truly means by the time you get home.

And you *will* get home. You've been living in a survival scenario your entire life. Through your wits, wisdom, and wherewithal, you've lasted up to this point, and you come from a long line of human beings who did a lot more with a lot less in worse conditions. You are that same creature. Even today, what folks in the developed world call an "outdoors survival situation" is just another Monday for people in less fortunate circumstances.

Remember You will survive. You will get home, and you'll have a great story to tell.

—Ben

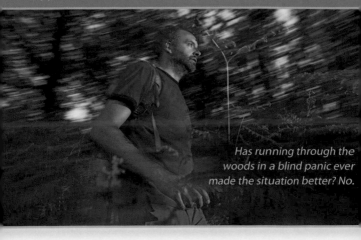

Has running through the woods in a blind panic ever made the situation better? No.

Prepare in Advance—Tell Someone Your Outdoor Plans You've likely heard this before, but it is the most important element to getting you home safely. Share your plans with someone you can trust to contact authorities if you don't return on time. Life-or-death survival situations are often a chain of failures, not one sudden disaster. Don't let this simple step be one of them.

S.T.O.P. The moment you realize you're in a survival situation can also be when your adrenaline makes things worse. Let the panic happen, but *stop*.

- **S**top, as in physically. Give yourself as much time as you need to calm down.

- **T**hink about what led up to this point.

- **O**bserve your current situation.

- **P**lan your next moves.

Use your brain before you use your body.

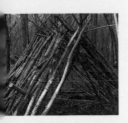

The 3-3-3 Rule A typical person can survive for three hours without shelter in dangerous conditions, three days without water, and three weeks or longer without food.

Know the Four - Shelter, Fire, Water, Food In terms of priority, first find or build a shelter, then make a fire, then source water, and finally find food. Why this order? Shelter will make it easier to build a fire, since you'll create a shield from the weather and, depending on the type of shelter, gather wood in the process. A fire gets your distress signal (smoke) into the air right away. Find water and you have a way to boil it at the ready. Food always comes last because you can go three weeks, or even longer, without it.

Depending on the situation, the order may change, but the point is to consider how one task can flow seamlessly into the next. This conserves time and energy.

Most Lost People Are Found in the First Two Days Most people who are lost in the outdoors are found within 48 hours. The odds are on your side. Survival, therefore, becomes less about what you do than what you don't do.

Cotton Kills/Cotton Equals Cold; Wool Equals Warm Consider your clothing choices before you head into the woods. Cotton clothing holds moisture against the skin. This keeps you cool in hot weather, but it can also lead to hypothermia at night. Wool, on the other hand, retains heat even when wet, and moves moisture away from skin. As a rule, wool trumps cotton. Synthetics have helpful properties, too. The point is to wear clothing that keeps you warm and dry at night, cool during the day.

On that note, keep clothing dry by removing layers when you're sweaty. Damp clothing is cold clothing when the sun goes down.

Whatever Litters Is Gold While litter is otherwise thought of as a nuisance, in a survival situation it is a blessing. Litter indicates the presence of human activity. A trail, road, campsite, or building could be nearby, increasing your chance of rescue. In a pinch, litter can also supplement your gear.

Two Is One, One Is None In terms of preparedness, if a type of gear is important to your survival, it is never enough to pack one of it. Bring two or more. For example, bring two packs of waterproof matches instead of one. Pair up a paper map with your GPS. Two knives, hatchets, or folding saws beat one. You get the idea.

Simplicity Equals Versatility Simplicity equals versatility when it comes to choosing gear. Reliable, basic tools that can be used in many different ways often outperform gadgets that merely claim to handle several tasks. For example, a sturdy knife will likely prove more versatile in the field than a multitool with 27 blade attachments. Apply that same philosophy to the rest of your gear. Simple is better.

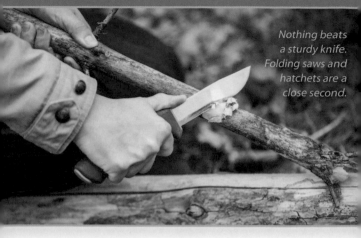

Nothing beats a sturdy knife. Folding saws and hatchets are a close second.

A Positive Attitude Is Your Best Tool Survival scenarios are extremely stressful. It sounds obvious, but you still need to stay positive however you can. Wrap yourself in prayer, positive affirmations, humor, games, music, reading material, or anything else to keep upbeat. In many real-world survival situations, the cynical wind up dead while their optimistic counterparts survive.

Knives Save Lives You will never understand this better than when your well-being depends on turning one of something into two: *Don't leave home without a knife.* However, some knives are better suited for survival than others. If you're reading this ahead of your survival scenario, skip the gimmicks and buy a knife with these characteristics:

- Fixed blade (the blade doesn't fold)

- Full tang (a single piece of metal forms the blade and the inside of the handle)

- A blade length from 3 to 5 inches

There are several options for knives beyond just these, and just as many opinions, but a decent survival knife will have all of the above characteristics. You know you're in the right territory when you're spending at least $100. Knives below that price point tend to skimp on the tang, which may mean your knife fails when put to hard use.

Folding Knives If a larger-size knife isn't your thing, or the thought of wearing a sheath on a long hike sounds uncomfortable, folding knives are a close second. While not as sturdy as fixed blade knives, they offer convenience and utility.

Folding knives ideal for survival will contain one or more of the following features.

- Blade length of at least 3 inches

- Handle material that is still "grippy" even when wet, such as G10 or Micarta. Lightly rubbing a handle with fine-grit sandpaper is an easy way to add even more grip, if desired.

- A blade that locks when open and must be unlocked to close. Of the several locking styles available, lockback knives are a great choice.

- Able to be opened with one hand, such as with assisted openers, automatics (where legal), and "flippers." This may save critical seconds during an important task, such as when making a fire.

Neck Knives Unfamiliar to some, but nonetheless handy, are neck knives. These small, fixed blade knives often consist of a single piece of steel. They're slipped into sheaths worn around the neck with a lanyard. Tucked beneath a shirt or jacket, neck knives offer quick accessibility and rugged designs. The downside is their small size, making them excellent secondary knives to a primary fixed or folding option.

Multitools Often referred to as "Swiss army knives" or "Leathermans" both specifically and generically, are another option. Treat them as secondary, supplemental knives. When push comes to shove, you need a solid knife that can take a beating. The moving parts on multitools are convenient but not nearly as durable.

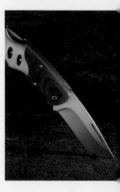

Even if the knife you carry into the outdoors doesn't meet these criteria, you're still better off with any knife than without one.

SHELTER

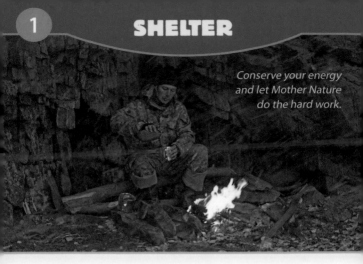

Conserve your energy and let Mother Nature do the hard work.

Clothing Is Your First Shelter The first line of shelter against the elements is your clothing. If you're appropriately dressed (in clothes that keep you warm and dry), skip creating a shelter and focus on finding a spot out of the wind. You're better off conserving your energy.

Layering clothing works along the same general principles, no matter the conditions. The base layer, closest to your skin (underwear counts here), mitigates moisture. The next layer traps or disperses heat. A weatherproof shell on the outside protects you from the elements. Add or subtract layers depending on your comfort.

However, if you're not able to withstand the elements with what's already on your back, you'll need to locate or make a shelter.

Where to Make a Shelter The ideal spot to make a shelter would contain the following elements:

- On level terrain, so rainwater doesn't flow downhill into your shelter

- Near a clearing, to increase the chance of being spotted by rescuers, but also sheltered from the wind/rain (for reference, prevailing winds typically come from the west, the same direction as the setting sun)

- Away from dead or dying trees, aka "widowmakers," and away from trees entirely if lightning is present

- A dry area

Clear out as much vegetation and debris from your shelter site as you can.

The Best Shelter Is the One You Don't Have to Make Sometimes Mother Nature can lend a helping hand. If something in your surroundings meets the requirements in the previous list, use it. The best shelter is the one you don't have to make. In April 2018, an Oregon truck driver lost in the woods crammed himself beneath logs to stay warm at night. He survived for four days before returning to civilization, as reported by CNN.

Smoke Out the Creepy-Crawlies Any time you make a shelter out of natural materials, you're going to be bunking with bugs that call leaves, grass, fallen branches, and other debris home. You can drive many of them out by wafting smoke from a nearby campfire into the shelter or by placing a piece of smoldering wood inside. Either requires careful monitoring so the shelter doesn't catch fire.

An Important Concept—Stay Off the Ground
No matter how you manage your shelter situation, keeping yourself off the ground is essential. That means putting a few inches between yourself and the dirt. The ground will suck the warmth out of your body, press moisture up against you, and expose you to bugs. If you don't already have a sleeping pad, make a "mattress" of leaves or grass. Pine needles are a great choice, too.

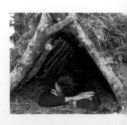

Four Simple Shelters Anyone Can Build Simple is smart. The more complicated a shelter is, the more likely it is to collapse, wear you down, or take up too much of your time. When building shelters, always try to conserve energy. The more you move, the more hydration you lose through sweat. Don't worry about mimicking the wilderness palaces you may have seen on the internet or TV. Knives, axes, and saws will make everything easier, although they're not required for these shelters.

Of course, a tent or other ready-made shelter is preferable to building one from scratch.

1) Super Simple—The Garbage Pile. The objective of the Garbage Pile is to provide quick shelter if you're injured, tired, or short on daylight. It's crude, but it works.

- Gather brush and other small debris into a pile. Dry is best.

- Build the pile as high and as wide as you can.

- Crawl inside the Garbage Pile feet first. If possible, wrap yourself in a tarp or survival blanket first.

- "Close the door" by putting something between your head and the outside, such as a backpack.

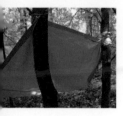

2) Set Up in Less than a Minute—A Tarp Lean-To. If you don't have a proper tent, a basic tarpaulin (or two) and some cordage can go a long way. There are two things to remember about tarps when purchasing them for survival purposes:

- Buy a high-visibility, orange tarp to make yourself more noticeable.

- A roll of 550 paracord is lightweight and convenient for tying down the tarp, but don't forget bungee cords. Bungees can be used for hundreds of tasks, and they make tying down a tarp easier, although they are heavier.

Tarps can be arranged in any number of ways, but the lean-to is the most basic and a good place to start, unless you have time to experiment.

- Tie two corners to branches at or above head level. The tauter the tarp can be made, the better.

- Tie the two remaining corners near to the ground, or stake them into the ground (use sticks if proper stakes aren't available), so that the tarp forms a 45-degree angle.

- If the tarp is too large to be practical for this design, make a tent with two 45-degree angles facing each other, tying the middle section at or above your head to branches. You can also make that middle support by leaning a log against a tree and draping the tarp across the sides.

When using a tarp, it is especially important to consider the wind. Point the "roof" of the tarp into the wind.

If you don't have bungee cords or paracord, use your shoelaces to tie the lean-to to branches, then stake the tarp to the ground using sticks. You can always untie the laces if you want to travel. Strips of clothing can work, too.

Even if you're unable to create a shelter with a tarp, wrapping yourself in a tarp to keep out the elements while you sleep is also a great alternative.

The downside of tarps is that they don't insulate, but they do offer terrific protection from the elements, enabling you to make a fire beneath them. If that's your plan, consider exactly where the fire will be made and where you will sleep before the tarp shelter is erected.

3) Got a Bit More Time and Energy? Try the All-Natural Lean-To.

This variant of the lean-to uses forest debris instead of a tarp. It takes more time and energy to create, but it works along the same principles. Building it will take at least an hour.

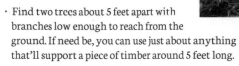

- Find two trees about 5 feet apart with branches low enough to reach from the ground. If need be, you can use just about anything that'll support a piece of timber around 5 feet long.

- Run a log or a thick branch horizontally between the branches on either tree at head level. Get as close to 180 degrees/level as you can. If available, secure the log with cordage to the trees.

- Stack logs or thick branches diagonally against the first log. Keep the logs/branches as close together as you can.

- Lay lighter branches against the logs. Keep adding layers of lighter and lighter debris.

4) The A-Frame.

An A-frame is a classic outdoor survival shelter. It follows the shape of a tent, but it's made from natural debris. It's also the most time- and energy-intensive shelter discussed here. Figure in at least a couple of hours of build time, as well as some healthy sweating. The objective is to create a frame out of thicker wood that you insulate with branches, leaves, grass, and other small plant material.

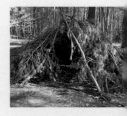

- Make three poles out of logs or thick branches (stripped down so they're single pieces of wood). Each pole should have a Y shape at the end. One pole should be longer than the other two. The longer one should be longer than you are tall. The other two should ideally both be 3 feet or so.

- Make a tripod, fixing the Y shapes together and facing the two shorter poles toward each other. Secure the tripod with cordage.

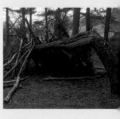

- Stack smaller logs and branches against the length of the tripod. Insulate with debris, such as leaves or grass.

- The more you secure the A-frame with cordage, the better.

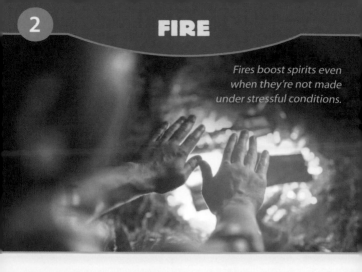

Fires boost spirits even when they're not made under stressful conditions.

Fire Is More than Flames Once your shelter is finished, making a fire is the next priority. A fire provides heat, of course, and offers a light during the night, but it also has many other functions. A fire does many things at once.

- Enables you to boil drinking water and cook food
- Keeps wild animals away
- Smokes out bugs in your shelter and in the air
- Dries clothing
- Provides a way to signal for help
- Gives you something to focus on
- Adds a companion

Matches and Lighters Beat Rubbing Sticks Together Modern methods of making fire *always* trump primitive methods. The latter are not covered in this guide because they take time and energy that you likely don't have. Stock up on waterproof matches, lighters, and resealable waterproof bags/containers instead.

Firesteels/ferro rods that throw sparks when scraped sit somewhere between the modern and primitive, but they are still far less reliable than matches and lighters, so don't leave home without the easiest way possible to make a fire.

Artificial Tinder While you can source tinder in the outdoors, premade tinder is highly recommended. If it can stay dry in a pack, light with minimal effort, and hold a flame for at least 30 seconds, it's good to go.

Buy or make tinder when you're stocking up on matches/lighters. A simple way to make tinder at home is to dip cotton balls into melted petroleum jelly. Store the tinder in a resealable, waterproof bag or container. Dry cotton balls minus the jelly also work.

A variety of weather-resistant firestarter products are available online for purchase, too. WetFire, for example, comes as a small cube that burns in almost any condition.

Natural Tinder When it comes to tinder sourced from Mother Nature, remember this general concept: anything combustible can become tinder if it's small enough.

If dry grass, leaves, bark, or sticks won't seem to work, cut them into small pieces or grind them into a powder. The increased surface area will amplify their combustibility.

Know Your Kindling—Feather Sticks One of the best forms of kindling is called the "feather stick." This involves cutting several narrow curls in a stick so that it resembles a bundle of feathers. These are added to the fire after the tinder gets going.

Rocks Are a Fire's Best Friend When you prepare your fire, placing rocks around the perimeter of the burn isn't just for aesthetics. Rocks hold heat. Carefully slip those rocks inside your shelter or sleeping bag, and you've got a great way to stay warmer at night while you sleep. Rocks the size of grapefruits tend to work the best for this purpose.

Dead Wood = You Alive Dead, dry wood is ideal for building fires. But if there isn't much nearby, look for fallen trees and low-hanging leafless branches for fuel.

Pass the Baton Split wood burns better than unsplit wood, but Mother Nature won't magically tackle this task for you. If you have a saw or hatchet, this is straightforward. If all you have is a knife, you'll need to "baton" the wood.

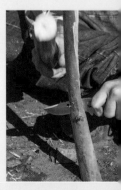

This involves beating the blade of the knife through the wood with another piece of wood. To get started, place the blade down on the piece of wood you want to cut. The blade should be longer than the wood it's placed against. Strike the spine of the blade with another piece of wood, using it like a hammer. Split logs, make kindling, or break down large branches with this technique.

Where to Make a Fire

- Beneath your shelter (in the case of tarps and lean-to shelters) or a few feet away from it
- Out of the wind and rain
- On dry ground
- Close to a source of fuel

Three Ways to Make a Fire When it comes to making a fire, no amount of instruction can replace practice. Matches and lighters are great, but the best tool for building fires under stress is experience.

1) Making the Basic Fire. This assumes conditions are decent and you're prepared with proper fire-making gear. In this respect, a survival fire isn't much different than an average campfire. There are a few considerations to keep in mind for the sake of efficiency:

- After selecting a spot for your fire, clear the area of debris.
- If available, place rocks in a circle around the spot where you're building your fire.
- Gather tinder and wood *before* starting the fire. Place these next to the spot your fire will be. You shouldn't stop to find fuel after you get the tinder going.
- Organize fuel into piles: tinder, twigs, sticks, big sticks, branches, and larger pieces of wood. The piles should all be within reach.
- Light the tinder, then add progressively larger pieces of fuel to the fire.
- Keep the fire going.

The challenge to keeping the fire going is that fuel will become farther and farther away as time goes on. Get creative to conserve energy. A long, single branch can provide you with almost every size of wood you'll need.

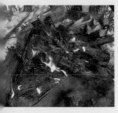

2) Make an Upside-Down Fire in Wet Conditions. There's no way around it: making a fire in wet conditions is exceptionally challenging. Prepare for several failed attempts. It's worth it to wait for better weather if you're too frustrated. At a certain point, you're wasting your breath.

- If it's raining or snowing, the first step is to create shelter for the fire to sit beneath.
- Clear the area of debris and create a platform of rocks or logs. You'll build your fire on top of this, keeping the fire off the wet ground.

- To find fuel for the fire, a core of drier wood can usually be found inside damp—but not waterlogged—wood, provided you baton or saw it out. Dead, dry branches can often be found low on trees, sheltered from rain and snow. Break down what you find into tiny, small, medium, and large pieces. Note that lots of kindling is required for an upside-down fire, so prepare more than you think you'll need.

- Now build an "upside-down fire" by crisscrossing the wood in order from largest to smallest (largest on bottom, smallest on top, like a pyramid). Place kindling at the top and light the tinder. This creates a self-feeding effect as the fire moves down the pile, drying out progressively larger pieces of wood.

- Feed the fire lots of air by blowing on it; this keeps the flames hot.

3) Making a Fire Without Matches/ Lighters: Here Comes the Sun.

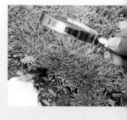

Should you find yourself without matches or lighters, light from the sun can be used instead. Yes, this really works, although the intensity of the sun needs to be quite high and the tinder exceptionally dry. It works best if the tinder is something artificial, such as a piece of paper. With that said, this is not an ideal way to start a fire, so don't leave home without your matches or lighters.

The classic way to do this is with a magnifying glass, but since you likely don't have one, some alternatives are:

- Binoculars; for this to work, you need to remove a lens to focus sunlight, but test your binoculars beforehand, as not all binoculars have removable lenses. If they do, the lenses unscrew, and you can then use them like a magnifying glass to focus the light.

- A clear bottle of water with the wrapper removed (position the bottle between the tinder and the sun).

- The polished, shiny bottom of an aluminum can (point it at the sun, then hold the tinder between the can and the sun).

The objective is to concentrate a single, tiny point of sunlight on the tinder. You'll have to experiment to get the angle right, but you'll know you've done it correctly when the tinder starts smoking. Add the smoking tinder to a waiting bundle of other tinder (dry grass folded in half is the classic choice), and then hold the bundle in your hands and give everything a gentle blow to get the flame going.

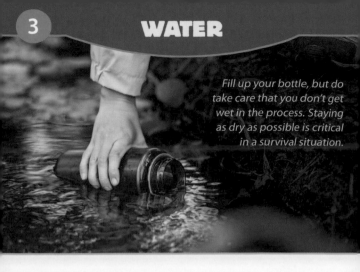

Fill up your bottle, but do take care that you don't get wet in the process. Staying as dry as possible is critical in a survival situation.

Water Is More Important than Food Staying hydrated will keep your mind and body sharp. You can't go more than three days without water, which is why it comes before food on the list of priorities.

Don't Ration Your Water Rationing clean water that's already on hand may seem like a smart move, but it hastens dehydration. Drink as you would normally to keep yourself primed while you search for other sources of water.

Think about it: Does it make sense to willingly muddy your senses at a critical moment if you know that most people are rescued within 48 hours? Also, you can't spill or lose water that's already inside you.

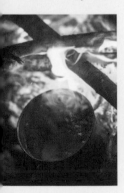

Making Established Water Sources Safe to Drink By default, assume that water found in lakes, ponds, streams, and rivers is dangerous to drink. It doesn't matter if the water is moving or standing—consider it all unsafe.

That said, you're in a great position should you find yourself near an established source of water. All you need to do is make it safe to drink. To do so ideally involves two steps:

- Filtering (a physical process) that removes organic materials, sediment, and most parasites and bacteria

- Purifying (a chemical process) that kills viruses, parasites, and bacteria

Filter first, then purify. Note that a dedicated survival product that filters may not require purification, although filtering by any means is always recommended prior to purification.

Filtering can be done several ways:

- A survival product, such as the LifeStraw or a filtered pump

- Cloth, such as socks, shirts, or bandannas (use in tandem with a purification method)

- Coffee filters (use in tandem with a purification method)

Following filtration, purification is up next:

- Boiling is the classic way to ensure safety. It's also easy to recognize when the water is safe, as most people are familiar with how to boil water. The water tastes best, too. This is the best choice. According to CDC recommendations, 60 seconds of a rolling boil is enough to kill the baddies unless you're at a high altitude, in which case you need to boil water for 3 minutes.

- Purification tablets, provided they are not expired and you *follow the directions on the package*. Don't wing it. (Note that the water will taste gross.)

- A UV-light device, such as the SteriPen.

Please remember to wipe up or disinfect any part of a drinking container that has come in contact with untreated water.

How to Find Water When There Aren't Established Sources When water isn't present as an established source, you're not out of options. Here are a few ideas.

Dew. One concept will be true no matter where you are: When temperature changes, so does water in the air. Air releases moisture when it cools, which means the mornings often will be full of dew.

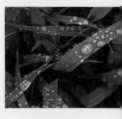

This is a prime opportunity for harvesting water. Like rain, fresh dew doesn't need to be purified before you drink it.

This is where the water-absorbing properties of cotton can actually help you. Run a T-shirt, bandanna, or other lightweight clothing through dew on low-hanging branches, in tall grass, or just above the ground. Squeeze what you gather into your mouth or a container. One trick is to tie a T-shirt around your leg and walk through tall grass. Regardless of how you do it, gathering dew is worth the energy.

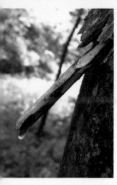

Tapping Trees. Tapping deciduous (i.e., not pine) trees works best in fall when sap (which can be consumed like water) is moving toward roots. Late winter and early spring can also work, too. If you get this technique right, you'll end up with a wilderness water faucet (albeit one that provides drips of water). Maple and birch are prime choices.

Before putting any holes into trees, observe your surroundings. Where is sap already dripping onto the ground? Look for snapped-off tree branches and listen for drips. If there aren't any, are any trees leaking sap down their trunks? You've found a candidate for tapping.

If you're lucky enough to find a drip, catch the sap with a bottle or container. It's generally safe to drink raw, but filter/purify it if you can.

To make your faucet:

- Using a knife, make a 33-degree upward cut into the tree's trunk about 2–3 inches deep. Twist the knife to create a small hole.

- Sharpen a small, stubby stick and place it into the cut so that the point facing you is angled downward.

- Water should drip off the end of the stick. You may have to wait several minutes for the drip to start, so come back to the stick later if necessary.

- Hold a bottle to catch the water. Wrap cordage around the trunk to hold the bottle in place.

This may take a few tries, even on the same tree. Go with mature trees for the best odds.

Rain and Snow. Rain and snow are obvious sources of ready-to-drink water, but there are a couple of pointers.

With rain, be strategic and purposeful about how you catch water. A well-placed tarp can act like a trough to fill smaller containers.

Snow should be melted in a container before it's consumed. Not only is this easier on your body, but it also separates water from debris in the snow.

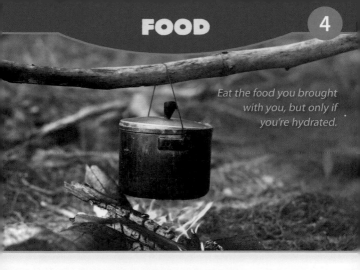

Eat the food you brought with you, but only if you're hydrated.

Food Isn't for Eating Good news! Seven out of ten adult Americans are overweight, according to the Centers for Disease Control and Prevention. This means your greatest caloric asset in a survival situation is already around your waist. You'll last at least three weeks before that reserve runs out.

It also means that food shouldn't be a concern in a survival situation. Foraging and hunting can be rewarding pastimes, but a survival situation is not the ideal time to try them out. The benefits may not exceed the costs.

First off, *every time you put something from the wild into your mouth, you increase your odds of becoming sick.* That's especially true if you don't have experience foraging and identifying wild foods. If you eat the wrong food, you'll likely get diarrhea and that can dehydrate you and kill you.

Second, consider how many calories it would take to source food. Harvesting wild foods is work. For example, 1 cup of dandelion leaves, a common source of survival food, contains 25 calories. How many calories would you burn gathering those leaves? How much more water would you need to drink for foraging and digestion? Is it worth it?

The answer is no. Inventory the food you already have on hand, and decide how you'll ration it. Since your calories are already inside you, use food to lift your spirits or soothe hunger pangs.

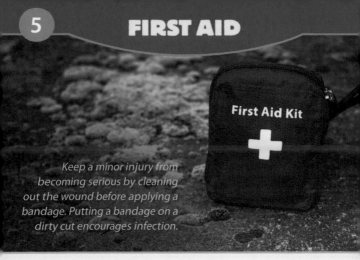

Keep a minor injury from becoming serious by cleaning out the wound before applying a bandage. Putting a bandage on a dirty cut encourages infection.

Remember This Word—Stabilize There's only one concept you need to remember for first aid: stabilize. Unless you're an MD, you won't be performing medical miracles in the field. Your goal is to keep the injury from becoming worse until help can arrive.

Cuts

- Stop the bleeding by applying pressure to the cut.

- If shallow, rinse the wound with clean water and a disinfectant If deep, do not apply disinfectant, as it can lead to later infection; instead, wrap loosely with dry gauze.

- Apply continuous, direct pressure with a bandage.

- If severe bleeding in the arms and legs won't stop with pressure, apply a tourniquet. This is a last-ditch technique, as tourniquets can kill the entire extremity.

Shock can be brought on by any number of factors, from trauma to an allergy. According to the Mayo Clinic, the signs of shock include:

- Cool, clammy skin
- Pale or ashen skin
- Rapid pulse
- Rapid breathing
- Nausea or vomiting
- Enlarged pupils
- Weakness or fatigue
- Dizziness or fainting
- Changes in mental status, such as anxiousness or agitation

If someone is in shock, cover them with a blanket, keep them still, have their legs slightly elevated, have them refrain from eating or drinking, and tilt their head to the side if they are vomiting.

Hypothermia is when the body loses more heat than it can create. It is a constant threat, as hypothermia can strike in any season (not just winter). For instance, sweat from clothing created during the hot day can become a hazard during the cool night. Hypothermia can lead to loss of consciousness and death. According to the Mayo Clinic, these signs indicate hypothermia:

- Shivering
- Slurred speech or mumbling
- Slow, shallow breathing
- Weak pulse
- Clumsiness/lack of coordination
- Drowsiness or very low energy
- Confusion or memory loss
- Dizziness or fainting
- Changes in mental status or behavior, such as anxiousness or agitation

Warm up and/or dry out to treat the onset of hypothermia. Get those wet clothes off of you, too. The sooner, the better, because your thinking will only become more impaired as the condition takes hold. That's why prevention is so important. Stay warm *and dry,* no matter the season.

Heatstroke is the opposite of hypothermia. It occurs when the body can't cool itself. According to the Mayo Clinic, the symptoms include:

- Skin that's hot to the touch
- Confusion, irritability, slurred speech
- Nausea
- Rapid breathing/racing heart
- Headache

Cool off immediately if you suspect heatstroke is setting in. Head to the shade, drink water, and remove any tight-fitting clothing.

Biting Insects like ticks, mosquitoes, and flies are annoying, carry diseases, and keep you awake at night. If you don't have bug spray, the best bet is to stay near your fire. Check yourself for ticks often, keep pants tucked into socks, and try to cover exposed skin when you're not moving. Biting bugs spread misery as much as anything else.

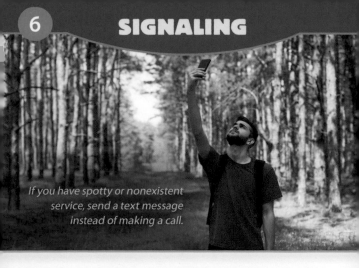

If you have spotty or nonexistent service, send a text message instead of making a call.

Signaling Is the One Thing You're Always Doing Signaling to rescuers is something that you should always be doing or always be thinking about because, odds are, that's how you'll get home.

Always ask yourself how your current task can pull double duty and make you easier to find. Could you build two fires instead of one? Could you build your shelter or pitch your tent closer to a clearing? Even if it's singing to yourself while you boil water, you're making extra noise, and that's worth something. It's all about increasing the odds in your favor.

Cell Phones/Smartphones Mobile phones are a lifeline—when they work. If reception is spotty, send a text message instead of calling. Not only will this save battery life, the phone will continuously try to send the message even if it doesn't go through right away.

If you have service on your smartphone but can't reach 911/emergency services through a phone call, use social media (especially Twitter) to send a distress message to many people at one time. If you can, send helpful pictures, too.

Keep your phone charged by packing spare batteries or power cells, or by bringing along dedicated survival products. I've tested and recommend the PowerPot. First, it's a pot that can boil water. Second, it's a charging station for your phone that runs on electricity generated by the water inside heating up. The water doesn't need to be boiling. This multipurpose approach is efficient and practical.

Portable solar panel rolls work well, too, but stay mindful of durability. Protective cases for the rolls should be rugged and able to take a beating without accidentally popping open.

Signaling to Aerial Searchers Make yourself as obvious to airplanes and helicopters as possible. Here are some suggestions:

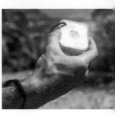

- Light a fire.
- Make your camp near a clearing.
- Write "SOS" in logs or rocks.
- Use a signaling mirror (a survival product) or other glass to reflect light toward an aerial vehicle.
- Burn trash, especially if it contains plastic or rubber, to create thicker, more noticeable smoke.
- Spread out a brightly colored tarp.
- Generally speaking, position materials that contrast with the surroundings. For example, a green tent could be pitched in a field of yellow flowers instead of a field of green grass.
- Stay in or near a vehicle.
- Launch flares.
- Deploy a smoke signal (a survival product).
- If none of these are options, get in a visible area and wave leafy branches.

A search plane may rock its wings back and forth in acknowledgment before leaving to get help. A helicopter will likely land or hover near you.

Audible Signals Here are a few suggestions for catching the ears of searchers on foot:

- Shouting
- Using a rescue whistle (a survival product)
- A car alarm or horn (if in a vehicle)
- Firing a firearm
- Slapping thick sticks against tree trunks or rocks
- Banging pots and pans together
- Using an air horn

Olfactory Signals An overlooked part of signaling is through smell. Burning plastic, rubber, or damp leaves can carry a stinky signal downwind. Don't discount this option.

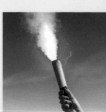

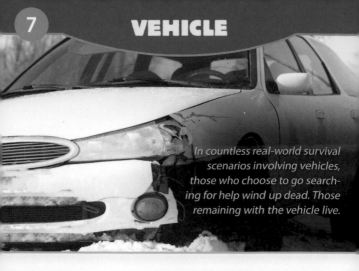

In countless real-world survival scenarios involving vehicles, those who choose to go searching for help wind up dead. Those remaining with the vehicle live.

Stay with the Vehicle Should your survival scenario involve you and a vehicle, you're in luck. Cars and trucks provide several survival necessities. For that reason, you're better off staying with the vehicle until you can get rescued.

Most of What You Need Is in the Vehicle Sticking with your vehicle has many benefits. It provides shelter from the elements, shade from the hot sun, a warm place to sleep, and an easy way to be spotted from the air.

The car itself has many survival-friendly features:

- Mirrors can be removed and used to signal aircraft or start fires.
- The horn and car alarm can be used to alert rescuers.
- Headlights and taillights can signal searchers in the dark.
- Everyday interior garbage and seat cushions provide a dry source of tinder.
- In a pinch, you can burn the tires for warmth and to create a thick smoke signal.
- Gasoline can be siphoned to use as an accelerant.
- Cigarette lighters can be used to light tinder.
- The radio provides weather updates.
- Vehicles with charging ports can keep cell phones charged.

Should you decide to abandon the vehicle, remember that you're also leaving all these assets behind.

Also, using jumper cables to light fires—either with sparks or by clamping a graphite/wood pencil—may seem like a good idea, but this could lead to a battery explosion and serious injury. You're better off using the vehicle's cigarette lighter or matches/lighters that you packed ahead of time.

*Moving usually makes
the situation worse.*

You're Better Off Not Moving Staying put is the best bet for rescue in a survival situation. Setting out on foot speeds up dehydration, expends energy, increases exposure to the elements, and is an easy way to get lost. You're also moving away from your last known location, which is where rescuers will logically start their searches. Even if more than 48 hours have gone by since your survival scenario began, you're better off not moving.

Sometimes, when there are two or more people involved, one person will go off looking for help while the other(s) stays behind. This is also inadvisable. There are many cases where a family member has left their children/partner behind in an attempt to seek help, only for the would-be rescuer to die. Again, staying put is nearly always the best strategy.

When to Move You *might* move for these reasons:

- To walk a road or trail you know leads to help
- To find cell phone reception
- To relocate to better shelter
- To source water
- To make yourself more visible to rescuers
- Something about your present location is unsafe

Moving should *only be done if it will improve your situation*. It's not enough to move because you get the itch to do so.

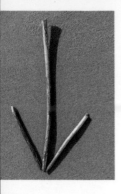

If You Move, Make It Obvious Before you move, leave some sort of signal indicating where you went. Common ways of doing this are a written note, rocks or sticks gathered to make an arrow, info carved into a tree, or a message dug into the dirt.

While you're on the move, mark your path in the most obvious way possible. Drag a thick stick or branch behind you, snap off branches, clear debris, drop debris, or simply shuffle your feet. Not only will this help searchers, you'll be able to find your way back to your original location if needed.

Also, if you can, walk in exposed areas. You'll be easier to spot from the air.

Document Everything Writing down notes about what you see and taking pictures of landmarks are excellent tools for navigating your situation, regardless of whether you move. If you lose your sense of direction or need to communicate by phone where you are, you have that reference available; your memory may not work so well under stress.

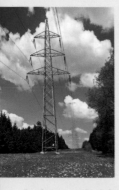

Power Lines and Water Usually Lead to Roads or People This is generally true, except in the most remote areas. In either case, there's also an old adage that says walking downhill will lead to people, safety, or "out" of the woods. There are too many variables in play to consider this sound advice. A better strategy is to ensure that you're heading in one direction and not in a circle. Use a compass, maps, landmarks, the sun, or stars to keep yourself moving in a single direction. This is not only practical; it keeps your mind occupied and reassured.

On that note, don't let a survival situation be the first time you look at a map of the area. Scout your location ahead of time on paper before you have to do it on foot.

Once You're Found After things settle down, keep in mind how helpful sharing your story can be to others. It's a personal decision, but many people never consider survival situations unless they hear about them from others. You just might save someone's life.